INDIA's HEALTH:

Problems and Solutions ©

Dr. S.K. Kajal

PREFACE

In the past few years the doctor-patient relationship in our country has deteriorated. Every other day there is news of violence against doctors, doctors going on strikes, allegations of irresponsibility by doctor in managing patients, over prized private hospitals, poor condition of government hospitals and many other things which has brought differences in the doctor-patient relationship. There is a perception in the society that medical profession has become business in this country. Even many doctors practice 'defensive medicine' just to protect themselves from any possible allegation. Due to this the patients don't trust their doctors and the doctors don't practice freely. This book outlines various problems in our health system and the possible solutions to these problems.

The quantity of doctors produced every year has increased but the quality has definitely decreased. This is because we have moved ahead in time but our medical curriculum and the pattern of examinations has remained the same as it was earlier. There is a separate section in this book addressing problems in the current undergraduate medical education.

Reservation in education system is a hot topic of debate among youngsters these days. So I have included a special section in this book addressing various issues with reservation.

Both positive and negative feedback is welcomed for this book. Do write to me - smilekajal92@yahoo.com

Table of Contents

TERTIARY HEALTH CARE

Tertiary Care in health system is defined as a specialized consultative care, usually on referral from primary or secondary
medical care personnel, by specialists working in a center that has personnel and facilities for special investigation and treatment. In simple language it is the highest level of health care available and ideally only cases referred from primary or secondary health care system are seen here.

Problem 1

There are more patients in almost all government run

tertiary care hospitals across the country than in a primary health care center. This is happening because there is no functional referral system operating in the country. Every individual directly comes to the highest center with symptoms which can be easily treated and should be treated in a Primary or Secondary health care center. For example, the outpatient department (OPD) of Internal Medicine is full of patients with symptoms like fever, cough, diarrhea, anxiety, etc. with history of such symptoms only for 2-3 days. Such patients waste time and energy of both doctors and the patients who actually need treatment in a tertiary care center.

Solution: Effective referral system

Every patient MUST follow the referral chain starting from Primary health center --> Secondary health center --> Tertiary health care center. A referral card must be issued to every patient before he/she reaches the next higher center. The higher center MUST ONLY see patients who have this referral card along with previous records of investigations and treatment received.

By the time a patient reaches the highest level of health care, he/she must have undergone all routine checkups which every patient must undergo regardless of any disease he/she is suffering from. Now some people may argue that a patient's condition might deteriorate by the time he reaches a tertiary health care center. Yes, it is possible but to prevent this - a doctor sitting in a Primary Health center (PHC) or Community Health Center (CHC) must be effective and intelligent enough to recognize the time to refer the patient to a higher center. And to produce such doctors we need to reform the undergraduate medical education from grassroots and the way to do this has been discussed later in the book. Strengthening of PHC and CHCs is also need of the hour to achieve such referral system. The ways to do this has been discussed in the next chapters.

Problem 2: Poor laboratory system

An effective and efficient lab system is a MUST for any hospital to provide best healthcare to the patients in today's world. Most of the government run hospitals in the country DO NOT have this. It is surprising that even in digital era, the technician has to enter the results of the investigations manually in a register to keep the records. Due to huge patient load, there is every possibility that some reports are missed. Another problem is that sometimes even the basic investigations are not being done either because the equipment is not available or it is not working. And then it takes months to get it repaired and during this time, the patient has to get that particular investigation from outside at higher price. Following is an example of working of lab system of one government run tertiary care hospital in Delhi. Things are not much different in other hospitals.

Suppose a doctor advises a patient to get his liver function test (LFT) done. If the patent has come to OPD, he needs to go to a sample collection room (and to find that room in such a big and unorganized hospital is really difficult). After finding that room, he needs to wait for his turn to give his sample because this place is overcrowded as all other places in the hospital. There is every possibility that by the time this person reaches the doorstep of this room, the time to collect sample is finished and he has to return home and come some other day or get the test done from outside. Let's assume that the person is able to give his sample. Now the next task is to find the place where he will get the result. This place is far away from the place where sample is collected and the result is available after 2-3 days. Now when the patient comes next time to collect his report, he has to find this place, wait for the technician to manually look into the records and then get the report back to the doctor's room where there are already 100 new patients.

Now let's suppose this patient is admitted in the ward and the senior doctor tells his post graduate or intern to send some blood investigations of this patient. Now there can be two situations

a) Its morning time and the doctor doesn't want report urgently – The patient should feel very lucky if this is the situation because now his sample will be sent from the ward to the laboratory by the nursing staff. (But nobody knows if the report is going to reach the ward or not!)

b) Anytime of the day and the doctor wants the report urgently (It's not doctor's fault here that he didn't send the investigation earlier. This situation may arise prior to start of a therapy which is required urgently if patient is deteriorating clinically). This is the worst situation for the patient because now he maynot get the investigation done inside the hospital because some of these investigations may not be available in the emergency lab of the hospital. So he's left with no option but to take the sample to a lab outside the hospital. And now there are men from different labs roaming about in the hospital wards to grab such opportunity, offering different prices and trying to take sample to their respective lab.

Another problem which may arise sometime is that the vials for ending the sample are not available in the hospital. Then first the patient has to buy these vials from outside and then get the investigation done.

Solution:

The first step to make laboratory working effective is digitalization of labs. This will solve maximum number of problems faced by both doctors and patients. If reports are entered into the computer and these computers in the lab are linked with computers in the wards or a common place in OPD, things will be so much easier.

Another step to make labs more patient friendly is to make separate building or select a common place to give samples and collect reports so that the patients don't have to run here and there. There can be different compartments inside this place (For example, one blood collection center, one urine sample collection center, one for stool, etc.) A separate compartment for samples coming from wards and a separate compartment for samples from OPD. The results of the investigations sent from wards should be linked directly to computers in the ward so that they reach the ward automatically and the doctor can see or print the report whenever he/she wants to. There should be separate report collection counter for OPD patients if it's not possible to provide computers in OPDs.

Problem 3: Poor infrastructure for Department of Radio diagnosis

With the advent of technology, this department has become very important in managing patients dealing with any specialty. Many tertiary care hospitals are surviving with only one CT scan machine and no MRI machine. This one CT machine is used for emergency as well as routine cases. And if due to any chance this machine becomes non-operational, then the patients are doomed because it costs less than Rs. 1000 to get a non-contrast CT in a government hospital while it costs around Rs. 5000 in private clinics (But this is NOT over-priced. It's just that poor patients who come to government hospitals cannot pay it. See discussion on Private health care in the coming sections). There are very less number of Ultrasound consoles. If such basic radiology equipment is not available, then one cannot even think of installing more advanced facilities like PET scan.

Solution:

Increasing the expenditure on health is the only solution to this problem. At least two CT scan machines to start with - one for emergency cases and one for routine OPD/ward patients. At least 5 Ultrasound (USG) consoles – two for emergency cases (USG is very commonly used investigation these days as it is non-invasive, quick, cheap and even confirmatory investigation of choice in many emergency cases), one for ward cases and two for routine OPD patients. And these days portable USG machines are available which can be used in emergency wards or even in other situations where patients are non-ambulatory. After this one can think of providing other facilities like echocardiography, Mammography, MRI, PET scan, etc. Again the results of these investigations should be available to patients online or should be sent digitally to the concerned doctor.

Problem 4: Long working hours of Resident doctors and poor working conditions

A first year post graduate works for 36-48 hours at one stretch in any clinical department and sometimes in working conditions which are neither good for the patient nor for the doctor. This point was highlighted very nicely in series of articles published in The Indian Express. One must google and read these articles to understand the depth of this problem. After reading these articles, one will understand that even basic facilities are not available in these so called tertiary hospitals. This is a loss to patients in terms that they have to buy stuff from outside. It is a loss to doctors as well because they cannot treat the patients despite knowing what to do but can't do it just due to lack of equipment. This situation is similar to a soldier who is standing in the battlefield without weapons.

Solution:

Increasing the workforce by increasing the number of post graduate seats. This will not only bring down the number of working hours but also bring an end to the trend of coaching classes going on in India (discussed later). Number of PG seats in a department are decided by the number of faculty members present in that department. So to increase the PG seats, one has to increase the number of faculty members and this is not a herculean task. There are so many doctors who are not promoted to the rank of professor or sometimes even associate professor just because of internal politics and poor administrative authority.

Improving the working conditions and making available the basic equipment/facilities to patients as well as to doctors is possible only by increasing the expenditure on health sector and by recruiting efficient hospital administrators. For Example, recruiting people who have completed Masters in Hospital Administration (MHA) for the post of Medical Superintendent (MS) and not just any doctor who is more concerned about managing patients rather than managing the whole hospital administration.

Problem 5: Providing everything free of cost

When the society is given everything free of cost, it's a natural tendency to misuse the facilities provided. Sometimes people roam about in the tertiary hospitals just because they think that they should have an ultrasound done for their complaints. Even if the doctor refuses in the first place, they pressurize the doctor to write them an ultrasound. This way they misuse the facilities which are provided for free.

Solution

Everything except emergency medical services should be

minimally prized. For example, OPD slip for Rs. 2 or Rs. 5, ultrasonography or other bigger investigations at a subsidized rate as well. This will not put much burden on the government as well. The doctors will also learn to use investigations judiciously. If everything is free, then doctors also know that everybody can afford anything and so he/she will develop a habit of ordering unnecessary investigations. There are some patients who are so poor that they cannot even afford these subsidized rates. Such patients can show their BPL (Below poverty line card) and avail everything for free.

The best solution to this problem is to enroll every citizen in compulsory health insurance scheme. This is discussed in later sections of the book.

RURAL HEALTH CARE

As on March 2012, there were 148366 sub-centers (SCs) and 24049 Primary health care centers (PHCs) and functional in the country.[1] A detailed statement of statistics (like population covered by each type of center against standard norm, health manpower, rural health infrastructure, demographic indicators, etc.) is released by Ministry of health and family welfare and is available online. Analyzing those statistics is not the aim of this section. The aim is to highlight the difficulties faced by patients, doctors and other health care personnel who are working in rural health system of India.

Problem 1: Poor Infrastructure and lack of basic facilities

Many Sub- centers and PHCs in villages do not have building of their own. Some are functioning in rented buildings while others are functioning in rent free panchayat or village society building. According to 2012 statistics, approximately 36% Sub-centers and 17% PHCs are in non- governmental building. This number may appear small but the bigger question is – Are all SCs and PHCs well equipped (whether in a government or a non-government building) in terms of medical facilities? The answer is no.

The basic investigations like Complete blood count, Serum electrolytes , Blood sugar, LFT, KFT are either not being done at all or some of these are done only once or twice a week. So if a doctor writes any of these investigations, the patient has to get it done from some non-authentic lab in the village. And most patients do not get it done because of high cost keeping in mind the low income of patients. Sometimes there is no electricity in the center and both patients and doctors suffer from this especially in the peak summer months. Many basic drugs go out of the stock towards end of the month and patient has to get them from outside. To some extent, the patients are also responsible for this because they take these medicines every other day (as if they are addicted to them) because they are free.

Solution:

Changing the infrastructure of every village is the first step to bring a change in the infrastructure of rural health centers. Villages need engineers equally, if not more than, they need doctors. Common problems of patients presenting in rural setup are infectious diseases. Where do these infections arise from? Poor sanitation, open sewage, garbage dumps, stagnant lakes/ponds, overcrowding – all these factors favor excellent growth of numerous microorganisms. The people can control only some of these factors if they maintain cleanliness around their houses (remembering the *Swacch Bharat Abhayan* of Government of India) But the major problem lies in the organization of the villages which can be provided only by the engineers who now days work only in IT companies in metro cities or look for big packages from foreign companies. Nobody blames them for not contributing anything to the society. Every other person blames doctors for not working in rural areas even when some are still working in whatever conditions available to them. All SCs and PHCs should have their own solar energy power generation capacity. Again, we need engineers for this purpose.

Problem 2: Doctors do not want to work in rural areas

Today's generation who opt for medical field is not at all interested in working in government hospital or more specifically rural government hospital. Even if government offers them a good amount of salary, most of them are still not ready to work. Why? Here's a brief explanation.

After finishing MBBS, almost all students try to get into some post -graduation (PG) course. Doing PG has become necessity these days because of changing preferences among patients and their family members. Most of the patients prefer going directly to a specialist which is surely wrong. But until and unless there is proper referral system (as described in previous section), this problem is going to persist. So after finishing MBBS, new doctors aspire for post-graduation. And after completing PG, they do not want to work in rural setting. This decision of theirs is justifiable.

Imagine a MD Internal Medicine doctor who starts working in primary or secondary health care. But what all can he do there? He has to prescribe only those medications which are available in the government hospital. And in rural setting there are very limited medications. He cannot manage medical emergencies properly (although he knows how to manage them) again because of lack of facilities and proper good quality medications. Ultimately he has to refer the patient to a higher center to save patient's life. So he is doing what a MBBS doctor would have done. So what is the use of him being a post graduate in Internal Medicine?

Take example of another specialties like General Surgery, Orthopedics, Ophthalmology or Otolaryngology. How are these surgeons going to work if they are not provided with good instruments, microscopes, etc. All that they had learnt during their post-graduation or during senior residency goes in vain if they cannot practice it.

And earning money is not everything. There is something called passion for your chosen specialty and exploring new dimensions in it which cannot be done in present working conditions of primary and secondary health care centers.

Solution:

There is a very important Department in medical colleges which can make huge difference in rural health system of our country. It is Department of Preventive and Social Medicine (PSM) or sometimes also called Department of Community Medicine. Doctors who are MD in PSM are expert in managing rural health or primary health care. They are expert in conducting various studies at primary level which help government in formulating various health schemes and programs. But unfortunately, they do not form the core of rural health system at present.

Some PHCs and CHCs are linked with Department of PSM of a medical college. The faculty, PGs, SRs and other staff members of this department perform excellent duty by visiting these centers, organizing various educational camps, and conducting various statistical studies. But other rural health centers which are not linked with any medical college are not at all in good condition.

The first step in improving rural health care is linking every rural center with the nearest medical college's Department of PSM. All heads of rural centers should either be MD from PSM or MD Family Medicine. Currently some hospitals do run MD family medicine course.

So at sub center level, only paramedical should be there. At PHC, a doctor trained in Family Medicine and at CHC, a doctor who is MD PSM should be the head of the center. Other specialty branches should start at CHC level.

Each state in our country is divided into districts which are then divided into tehsils which are further divided into blocks. Each block has many villages. To make a perfect hierarchy of health care, one district should function as one unit. Presently there are PHCs in villages which are linked to a CHC in a block or tehsil which are then linked to a district hospital. But the problem is that there is not major difference in the services provided sub district level and District level. There are only few hospitals in a state which provide tertiary care and every district or sub district hospital refers the patents to these hospitals when needed.

To make our government sector more efficient, every district hospital should be converted to a tertiary care hospital which should then be linked down to upgraded sub district hospitals by well-equipped ambulances. So there will be Primary, secondary and tertiary care hospital in each district which will function as one unit.

PRIVATE HEALTH CARE

Only **problem** for patients is High cost:

Now that we have understood that government health care sector is not providing the standard of care needed for patients as well as doctors, both of them look towards private health setup in the country which is far better and covers majority of the health services in India. But there is one problem for patients who want to go to a private hospital for treatment or just a routine checkup and that is Cost. A laparoscopic cholecystectomy which is done for free in government hospital (if all instruments, drapes and sutures are provided by government), costs around 15-30,000 in smaller cities, between 30,000 to 50,000 in big cities and may even cost 1 lakh in premier private medical institutions.

But just think that who provides for this cost? Nobody except the doctor who has opened up his clinic or the hospital authorities. With the money which the doctor earns, he/she has to pay the junior surgeon, the anesthetist, other hospital staff members, the electricity bills, other minor bills, the taxes, and then he has to save something for himself and his family just like any other common person. After 2 years of pre medical, 5 and half years of MBBS, 3 years of post-graduation, 3 years for Mch/DM or 3 years of senior residency, and then investing money to open up a well-equipped clinic/hospital - can't a doctor ask for Rs. 500 as consultation fee? Some people may still think the answer should be No because the doctor charges 500 but spends only 15 - 20 min or sometimes even less in normal private OPD. But people don't know that this doctor has spent 13 years (and this is without drop outs and spending more years studying and trying to get seat at each level – MBBS, MD/MS, Mch/DM) of his life to make a correct provisional diagnosis, order the right investigations and prescribing the correct treatment in just 15 minutes. Just imagine how many cases he/she must had seen and then studied about them while working as junior in his/her past to be able to do what he is doing in the present.

Another justification for high cost is the equipment. To open a full-fledged Eye hospital, a doctor needs at least Rs. 1 crore. This is because if he wants to provide the best care, he should have all the equipment required for opening an eye care hospital. In case of General surgeons, he/she has to spend lakhs of rupees just to get the right instruments. Where will a doctor, who has just finished his studies and want to practice independently, bring this money from? This is possible only if this doctor belongs to a very rich family or he takes loan from bank which he then pays back with interest if his practice goes well. Another example of the amount of investment required in setting up a private Radio diagnosis clinic is beyond mentioning as even the government does not have enough money to provide CT scans and MRI machines in minimum desired number in all tertiary care hospitals.

Even if a doctor is in non-surgical branches like MD Internal Medicine or MD Pediatrics which do not require big set-up, he/she takes consultation fee for his hard work which he has put in all those years to reach that position.

The society and news channels only point out at doctors as overpriced. What about other things which are clearly overpriced? On number one position are fast food chains where people spend lavishly and happily and when they come to see a doctor because of their bad eating habits, they call doctor as overpriced, greedy, and what not. People spend thousands of money to stay in a good hotel where they use room facilities like ACs, fridge, LCD, washrooms etc. but they call it overpriced when their patient is admitted in an ICU where there are ACs, equipment to keep the area sterile, ventilators, etc. whose investment cost is way more than those hotel rooms.

There is no denial that some doctors might be overcharging. But most doctors ask for genuine price if the above stated factors are taken into consideration. There are always two types of people in every profession – The good ones and the bad ones. There are good shopkeepers and bad shopkeepers, good politicians and bad politicians, good teachers and bad teachers, good police officers and bad police officers, good clerks and bad clerks, good engineers and bad engineers, good lawyers and bad lawyers, good actors and bad actors, good singers and bad singers, etc. Likewise there are good doctors and bad doctors. But the problem is that our media mostly talks about the bad ones. And a perception is made in the society that all doctors are like that.

There are many doctors who earn in good amount as well as help poor sections of the society in getting the best possible medical care. Many private hospitals/ private practitioners set up camps in rural areas for free without compromising the quality of health care. Our media must talk about these good ones because there is a chance that the bad ones may also become the good ones.

Solution:

First step towards reducing the health care cost is increasing the percentage of GDP spent on health and making government hospitals as equipped as private hospitals so that majority of the Indian population which lives in rural areas can avail best medical services at highly subsidized rates.

The cost of the private sector will always remain high because they provide the best medical care in our country. There are some things which are too overprized but they can be curbed if some regulations are set by the government. The only thing which private hospitals / doctors can do is setting up camps (without compromising the quality), reserving some beds in their wards for poor patients, organizing free OPD day in a week, public –private partnership etc.

The only sector left which really needs to do something to increase the quality and reduce the burden of private medical care on middle and lower class population is government sector. As stated above increasing the percentage of GDP on health should be the first step. Then comes the proper referral system (discussed earlier) – this will reduce the wastage of resources in tertiary care hospitals.

Another initiative which the government must take is 'Compulsory health insurance for all'. This step will lead to decrease financial burden on patients especially in case of emergency. Let the insurance company pay its client's cost directly to the doctor or hospital involved in the treatment. In this way patient will get the best treatment without worrying for money and the doctor will get his fees for his hard work. Developed nations like United States pay utmost importance to health insurance. They have various insurance plans according to their needs. There are low, middle and high premium plans offered to the population and services differ accordingly. Similarly we can formulate insurance plans depending upon needs of our population. Some insurance plans can also serve as a check on doctors who ask for unnecessary investigations just to make money.

EMERGENCY MEDICAL SERVICES

A common scene shown in Indian movies is that when a patient is brought in emergency department of a big private hospital, he/she is denied of any treatment because his family cannot bear the cost of the hospital. There is no denial that this does happen in some private hospitals. But again the hospital is not at fault here because the present system in our country does not give financial security to patients in case they land up in an emergency room. The hospital is bound to take money for the services it provides; be it before the treatment or after the treatment. But obviously denying the treatment is not right in any way.

The only way to rectify this situation is – 'Compulsory Health Insurance for all' as discussed earlier. The doctor and patient should not worry about the money especially in case of emergency. Let the insurance do its work.

A good emergency care is far away from the reach of majority of the Indian population. A well-equipped emergency room must be set up in every block of the country which should be linked to a tertiary care hospital by an ambulance which is not just a vehicle but a mobile emergency vehicle equipped with majority of emergency care needed by the patients. For example, an ECG machine, Automated external Defibrillator, portable ultrasound machine, IV drips, cannulas, emergency medications, etc.

UNDERGRADUATE MEDICAL EDUCATION

There are 143 recognized government medical colleges in India offering 20, 885 MBBS seats. If number of private medical colleges and other medical colleges which are not yet recognized (but only permitted for intake of students) are added to this figure, the final figure is 398 medical colleges and 52, 255 MBBS seats (as of April 2015). [2] The curriculum for teaching MBBS is vast which makes the course duration of 5 ½ years.

Problem 1: Duration of the course and pattern of teaching

Many students do not opt for medical stream after 10th standard just because of this. The main reason for this long duration of MBBS is unnecessary lecture schedules. Many lectures are repeated just for completing the number of hours allocated in the present curriculum. At undergraduate level, Ophthalmology and Otorhinolaryngology (ENT) have been given 1 year of duration which is unnecessary because these are highly specialized fields and what an undergraduate needs to learn in these fields can be completed in 6 months duration. According to the new trend, the lecture series for major clinical subjects (Internal Medicine, General Surgery, Obstetrics and Gynecology, Pediatrics) starts in 2nd year when the student is still learning about basic clinical sciences like Pathology and Pharmacology. This is again unnecessary because it takes up the time which could have been used to complete the syllabus of basic clinical sciences which make the cornerstone of whole MBBS and secondly, most students do not bother to read final year subjects in 2nd year (because 2nd year itself is very vast and very important) which leads to complete wastage of time spent in those major clinical subject classes just for the sake of covering up attendance.

Solution:

The first two years of MBBS should be completely dedicated to learning of Basic clinical subjects i.e. Anatomy, Physiology, biochemistry, Pathology, Pharmacology, Microbiology, Toxicology, Medical Ethics, Genetics, etc. The lecture schedule should be concise and without repetition. For example, if immunology has been taught once in biochemistry, there is no need of teaching the same thing again during lecture series of

Pathology or Microbiology. This needs departmental co-ordination.

The next two years of undergraduate medical education should be spent entirely in the hospital. The theoretical lecture schedules should be minimum and there should be more emphasis on clinical history taking and examination methods to diagnose a condition and its basic treatment. The detailed theoretical part of it can be read by students themselves from their textbooks.

The third year should comprise of 8 months of clinical rotations -

2 months each in Internal Medicine, General Surgery, Obstetrics and Gynecology and Pediatrics. The last four months should be divided among short subjects (short at undergraduate level!) like Ophthalmology, ENT, Dermatology and Orthopedics and Psychiatry. This year should emphasize on theoretical knowledge and clinical history taking and examination methods.

The final year should include 2 months each in Internal Medicine, General Surgery, Obstetrics and Gynecology and 1 month in Pediatrics. The next three months should be divided among short subjects like

Orthopedics, Radiology and Anesthesiology. This year should not only emphasize more on clinical history taking and examination methods but also basic treatment of common conditions encountered by a MBBS doctor.

The next 8 months should emphasize on practical procedures like taking out blood samples, inserting cannula, setting up an IV line, giving injections, various types of fluid taps, suturing, assisting in surgical procedures and many more. In these 8 months, the students should be rotated for 1 month each in Internal Medicine, General Surgery,

Obstetrics and Gynecology and Pediatrics. The next 2 months should be spent learning basics of Community medicine (including field trips, visiting primary health care centers, etc.) The next 1 month should comprise of clinical posting in one of the short subjects of student's own choice and the last 1 month in any subject which student likes.

If you calculate all this, it makes total duration of MBBS 4 ½ years including training for basic procedures which a MBBS doctor should know. The examinations can be adjusted in between this curriculum if we go into more details.

Problem 2: Subjective Pattern of Examination

The way a student gets tested in a medical college is by asking him to write long answers which he/she had crammed one or two nights earlier. There are no practical based questions. There are some fixed questions which are asked year after year. Every batch comes, crams the answers to these questions, passes and then forgets. In this way undergraduate students do not come to know about the art of using their theoretical knowledge in real medical situations. For example, every first year student must know how to draw brachial plexus for anatomy exam. Everyone makes different mnemonics to cram the names of nerves in it. If at all the question comes about brachial plexus (there is a high probability of getting a question from brachial plexus as it is a 'very important' topic for anatomy exam), all students draw it correctly. But if they encounter a patient with injury to one of the nerves of brachial plexus, very few will be able to recognize it because they were never asked the question in that way (or never taught that way).

Moreover, these subjective papers are checked by different teachers (obviously one person can't check thick 150-200 answer sheets in a limited time period) and there is no fair evaluation even if the quality of questions is good. Some teachers give marks according to the number of sheets filled by the student without even looking at the content. Most of the time questions asked are long or short answer types like the ones students get in high schools. There is no difference between the quality of questions asked in high school and professional medical college.

Solution:

Just look at the quality of questions asked in United States Medical licensing Examination

(USMLE). Each question makes the subject more interesting. The student comes to know about the actual application of the topic he has studied. Every question has clinical implication even if it asked from pre and para clinical subjects like Anatomy, Physiology, Biochemistry, Pathology, Microbiology, Pharmacology, etc. The student understands that studying and understanding these subjects is as important as studying clinical subjects because they form the pillars on which the whole medical field stands.

So the solution is to make a uniform evaluation process,

similar to USMLE, all over the country. The only difference will be that the emphasis will be on diseases or case scenarios which are common in India rather than in USA. One main exam (objective pattern and clinically oriented) at the end of first two years which will cover all basic sciences and another similar pattern exam at the end of course which will consist of all clinical subjects. These exams should be conducted all over India to bring uniformity in quality of doctors produced each year. These will be similar to Step 1 and Step 2 (clinical knowledge) exams of USMLE. The scores obtained in these exams should be used for entry into post-graduation course so that a student does not waste his time and energy in coaching institutions which help them in cramming 19 MBBS subjects and then they are tested in just 3-4 hours of so called post graduate entrance examination which has the poorest quality of questions possible. At present, no weightage is given to how a student had performed during MBBS, whether he/she was involved in any research project or not, whether he/she did some extra-curricular activities or not, or if he/she has good communication skills to deal with the patient.

The practical aspect of the curriculum should be tested in the same way as it is conducted by different universities in present times, that is, conducting viva and other practical procedures in pre & para clinical subjects and allocating cases in clinical subjects along with other procedural and instrumental viva.

Another popular method of evaluation is Objective Structured Clinical Examination (OSCE) in which a candidate is assessed on different stations and each station has a very specific task (e.g. Evaluation of a simulated or sometimes a real patient, an interpretation of any graph, identification of any lesion shown in the picture and answering the related one word question, etc.). OSCE is more relevant during practical examination. It is good to hear that many colleges have started using this evaluation practice during practical examinations.

Problem 3: Doctors as teachers

Many times a lecture which is scheduled to be held at a particular time does not take place because the teacher cum doctor was busy in some other academic/clinical activities. This happens mostly during lectures for clinical subjects. It's not doctor's fault. She/he has many other important responsibilities than taking an undergraduate lecture. Moreover many doctors feel it as a burden to teach undergraduate students simply because they don't have interest in teaching. They just want to focus on patient care. And when these doctors are forced to prepare and take a lecture, they do it half-heartedly resulting in wastage of their own as well as student's time. Such lectures are often known as 'boring lectures'. It's not the doctor's fault that he made the class boring. It is just that he doesn't like teaching and thinks it as a burden in his professional life. Moreover he/she is not getting any extra pay as compared to other non-teaching faculty/doctors working in the same medical college cum hospital.

Solution:

Recruit only those doctors for teaching in a medical college who have interest in teaching. When such teachers take a class/lecture, it can never be a boring class. Every student must have experienced this. Out of 10 lectures taken by different teachers, there are only one or two which are very interesting and every student in the class listens to the teacher. These are the teachers cum doctors who have passion for teaching. They do not take it as a burden. There should be proper division of labor between the teaching and non-teaching faculty (E.g. Give less ward duties to the teaching faculty so that they can engage themselves more for theoretical as well as practical classes) In this way everyone will be paid equally and there are very less chances of ego problems and intra departmental conflicts.

Problem 4: Internship

One extra year for training was designed to make medical students familiar with the hospital working and teach them various procedures which a medical graduate must be familiar with. Students used to take internship seriously a long time ago when the mad race for getting a post graduate seat was not a common trend. These days many students just leave the internship training just to study and get a post graduate seat without wasting another year preparing for it. Actually it is not their fault. It has become compulsory these days to get MD/MS degree so that one could survive in the competitive environment. This issue has been discussed later in the book.

Here the main concern is that at some places interns are made to do things which they are not supposed to do. For example, transporting samples or collecting sample reports, doing 24 hours duty, sending an intern for some personal work of a post graduate. According to the MCI (Medical council of India) internship guidelines [3],

5 (iii) 'an intern is not required to transport samples or collect reports of the patients (except in emergency situations)'

5 (vii) 'The intern shall not work consecutively for a period of 24 hours'.

There is no regulation on how much an intern should work. Interns working in medical colleges in Delhi and other reputed medical colleges work in excess while Interns in most of other medical colleges work below the required standards (talking about working hours). These days some students take externship in hospital nearby their permanent residential place where they do not go at all or work for very less hours. It's not their fault because, as stated earlier, it has become more of a compulsion these days to have a post graduate degree. So until and unless the whole curriculum is not transformed into something new (or 4 ½ year course as described above which already includes training in basic procedures), the internship training program will not be balanced in the whole country.

Solution:

Again no individual is at fault. The interns are made to collect reports because even big government hospitals in the country do not have efficient laboratory system which timely sends back the reports at correct places in hospital. Every lab should be linked to every ward/OPD of the hospital electronically so that one can check the status of patient's reports just by clicking a button whenever one wants to and without even leaving his/her ward duty roaming here there to collect report which is a total wastage of time and energy.

The interns are made to do 24 hour duty in some departments in some hospital because of less manpower which is a major issue in medical field (discussed later). But sometimes interns are made to do 24 hours even in the presence of manpower in the department just to make him/her stay. It is the duty of interns to talk to the appropriate authorities if such things happen.

If the medical curriculum proposed in solution to problem 1 is followed all over the country, there is no need for extra one year of internship and bothering about unnecessary duties and getting a post graduate seat. This is the best solution to eliminate the difference in working hours and conditions of Interns in different hospitals of the country.

The history of providing reservation to the 'oppressed class' of society goes back to pre-independent era. It was started for very genuine reason. There is no denial in the fact that this class of people had been suppressed by the upper class for centuries. The division of society in four main castes (Brahmins, Kshatriyas, Vaisyas, and Shudras) was done most probably for effective division of labor in the society. But it was not told to people that a person can change his so called caste just by doing the work of other caste. It was not taught to them that the caste of a person will not be decided by the family in which he/she was born. So people started believing in the fact that a child born in a particular caste will live with that caste forever. It was possible that if a person from lower caste became educated, then he would be counted among the Brahmins. Or if he chose to become a warrior, then he would be counted among Kshatriyas. Or the other way round, if a person from higher caste did not perform the duties assigned to that caste then he would be counted among the caste involved in performing other duties. But all this did not happen. What happened, as we all know, was that if a person is born in a particular caste will live with that caste forever. And due to this reason the people belonging to the lower caste were suppressed for hundreds of years. They did not get education, they were denied any good job opportunity, there was practice of untouchability, they were denied entry into any religious place ; in short, they were looked down as worse than slaves.

So initially reservation for these lower and deprived classes was necessary. It has helped many families in ways which their ancestors could not even think of. Just think of a family in which all previous generations had been working as cobblers and then the present generation has family members like a teacher, an engineer, or even one doctor. This happened because the present generation was able to study somehow and they had benefit of reservation. Now no one in the future generation of this family will have to work as a cobbler and everyone will contribute to the country's progress and economy.

But if reservation is so beneficial, then why is there so much hostility towards it and towards people belonging to reserved categories? Because there is no limit to it. There is no stop point.

Taking the example of same cobbler family mentioned above– now that the present generation has people working at good positions, it would be unfair to give reservation to kids of these people. A doctor of this family ('A') is the first doctor in his entire generation, but still he is a doctor and will now be counted in the society among all other non-reserved category doctors who may be having doctors in every generation. He might be earning less as compared to other doctor ('B') whose parents or even grandparents were also doctors but he has the same responsibility. Now 'A' has the opportunity to send his kids to good school, provide them as much facilities as he can, make them self dependent and send them to good college. All these things will also be done by 'B' whose earlier generations were also doctors. 'B' may still be having an upper hand in providing good facilities but this difference is a minor one and cannot be equalized by providing reservation to kids of 'A' just because 'A' belongs to a lower caste.

All non-reserved families are not rich families. If we keep on giving reservation to family 'A', then this will give undue advantage to this family over non reserved non rich families. These are the families which have developed maximum grudges against policy of reservation. To prevent this from happening, reservation has to stop at some point.

Solution:

Abolish caste based reservation because although maximum population of poor, deprived and needy people still belong to lower castes but such people are present in every caste. Giving reservation only to those belonging to lower caste is NOT justifiable.

After demarcating a line on the basis of family income and

quality of life (this is for government to decide that what should be that demarcating index), reservation should be provided. This should be different for rural and urban India because a person earning Rs 15,000/month in a rural area may be able to survive and provide genuine facilities to his kids but living with this amount in a big city and supporting a family is very difficult. So the rural family in this case may not fall under reservation policy but the urban family might. (This is completely a hypothetical example)

The period for which reservation is provided to a family must be fixed. Again taking the example of cobbler family. Its very rare possibility that the cobbler's kids will suddenly get such good opportunities and facilities that they get admission into a medical college and become a doctor, despite having an extra advantage of reservation. In most of the cases, the process is gradual. This cobbler's kids (2nd generation) will study most probably till 8th, 10th or maximum 12th standard because of different reasons (poor studying environment at house, financial reasons, lack of motivation, poor health etc.) Suppose if one of the cobbler's child studies till 12th standard, then he/she can apply for some job in government sector with an advantage of reservation and he doesn't have to work as a cobbler like his father. Now this government employee's kids (3rd generation) will get better opportunities than the previous generation and if they work hard and take advantage of reservation, then there is a high probability that someone will land up into a good professional college. This should be the stopping point. Once this happens, the next generation should not get the reservation. Or another thing which can be done is that the next generation children (that is, children of 3rd

generation who landed in a professional college) will come under reservation policy but they have to get above 50% (same as eligibility cut off in most exams for general category children) and NOT 40 %-45% as opposed to that required by 2nd or 3rd generation children. But after this NO RESERVATION AT ALL. So reservation policy must only be up to 3rd generation or maximum 4th generation with some changes. (All this reservation MUST NOT be based on caste from beginning itself)

Another possibility is that the government employee's children are not able to get into any professional college and instead they land up again at the same post as their father/mother (i.e. a government employee at a lower post). In such case, whether reservation should be given or not can be decided on the basis of present economic condition of the family.

So it took 3- 4 generations to transform a reserved category family to a non-reserved category family (i.e. from a very low earning work like that of a cobbler to high/average earning work like a doctor or other professional or a government employee above demarcating index). This means approximately 100 years; which implies that if a demarcating index is used today to give reservation, then it will take 80-120 years for bringing all families below it to unreserved category.

If this would have been thought when reservation was started, reservation would have been on the verge of end now.

But instead caste based reservation was chosen. Every other day members from new caste proclaim to be minority and deprived and demand of reservation. This adds numbers to those taking reservation. If this continues, then reservation is not going to end even in the next 100 years because same families will keep on taking reservation as their birth right because they were born in some lower caste and other castes will keep on demanding reservation.

The above example of following generations to end reservation is not possible practically but we can draw two important conclusions from it. First, Reservation is necessary to pull out people from poverty and give them better opportunities. Secondly, reservation should not be caste based. It should only be on the basis of economic condition of present generation family.

If a stopping point is chosen, then the number of families which need reservation will decrease gradually and finally a day will come when every Indian is self-dependent and he/she will not ask for any reservation to move ahead.

Special note – Punjab has the highest number of scheduled caste population in India (approximately 32%). This means 32% of Punjab's population is eligible for reservation in education, jobs, promotions, etc. But the irony is that Punjab is one of the wealthiest state of this country (NRI money!!) Some people contributing to this wealth also belong to these 32%

but still they are eligible for reservation only because we follow caste based reservation. Had we been following 'demarcation index' based reservation, this number would have been decreasing every year since many SCs would now be not eligible for reservation.

Reservation should be given only till entry into graduation course. Once a student enters a college, he/she gets same opportunities as others. It doesn't matter whether he/she is from a reserved category or unreserved category. Every student attends the same classes, attends the same lectures, gets the same practical exposure, and has to pass the exams with same minimum passing marks as required by all students. Then why is there reservation while seeking entry into a post-graduation program? There occurs no partiality except when done personally by a faculty member or other member or college staff or even by fellow student sometimes. There is law to protect students from such atrocities. No one will have courage to do such thing again, if even one student files a complaint of any such incidence. But our students don't have courage to do so. They are scared of failing in the exams if they complain against that faculty member. But they don't know that the law can 'fail' that person from his/her job, if found guilty. The categorization of reserved/unreserved should end once a student enters a college. Even if reservation is given in post-graduation, then why in jobs, promotions?

Some people may argue that reserved candidates do not have enough money to go to coaching classes required to clear post-graduation entrance examinations. To state the truth, coaching classes are a big hoax in this country (especially coaching for medical post-graduation). Their business will end automatically once the examination system of this country is modified.

Ending the reservation all together suddenly is not the solution. It has to be ended but gradually by the taking into consideration above points.

POST GRADUATION

Almost every doctor who graduates in today's time wants to pursue a post-graduation course because there are limited options for a doctor who has only MBBS degree. He/ She can work as medical officer in rural health care which is not in good condition as described earlier or he/she can setup a private clinic in village or small town. It is difficult for a doctor in a metropolitan city to survive if he/she has only MBBS degree as people in these cities go directly to a specialist (Again the fault is lack of referral system).

So every year lakhs of students appear for MD/MS exams which offer a few thousand seats. In a race to get into a post-graduate (PG) course, undergraduates tend to neglect practical aspects of their training and focus only on solving multiple choice question books and joining various coaching institutes.

Problem 1: Less number of PG seats

Every year the number of students who appear for PG exams increase but the number of seats either remain same or sometimes even decrease. The number of PG seats in any department of a medical college depends upon the number of faculty members. If any faculty member of a department resigns or gets retired the seats will decrease by one or two for each faculty member if that position of is not filled up. Less number of PGs in a department of a tertiary care hospital leads to overburden of PG students which leads to frustration which leads to impaired personal life as well as impaired patient care. It has been proven in a study that if one misses one night sleep, then his/her brain functions similar to that of a legally drunk person. Now imagine the condition of PGs who work continuously for 36-48 hours. This is one of the main reason which leads to violence inside the hospital premises because every patient expects best care but the doctor is not able to provide this care due to overburdening and patients do not understand this. So actually it is no one's fault.

Solution:

It is very important to increase number of PG seats because it will lead to better patient care and better personal life of doctor. To do this, allot more number of PG students to faculty members or if that is not possible, then increase the number of faculty members by giving timely promotions to senior residents and Assistant Professors.

Problem 2: Frequent attacks by patients on Resident doctors

Every now and there is news of a doctor being beaten up by patent's attendants who accuse the doctor for their patient's death because according to them the doctor did not provide adequate medical care. This is the story in almost every news. And the interesting part is that the news shows doctor as the villain in almost every case. I have not seen or read any news till now which shows that the doctor was not at fault. Obviously the news channels are not the court of law. But if they cannot show the real story or if they do not know the real situation which led to the present condition, they have no right to accuse the doctor every time and destroy his career. They do not have any right to decide that the patient is always on the correct side.

In most of the situations, the patients are not wrong and the doctor are not the one who caused harm. So if both doctor and patient are right, then who should be blamed? There must be someone or something which leads to misunderstanding between the two which then has serious consequences. Few of these things are as follows –

a) Patients overburdening a tertiary care hospital (because referral system not followed in this country)

b) Overburdened doctors (due to lack of manpower)

c) Miscommunication

d) Political interference

e) Patients expecting miracles

No doubt that there are doctors who talk very rudely to the patient. There are doctors who suck out money from patients un-necessarily. But as mentioned in earlier, there are good ones and bad ones in every field. The problem is that our media loves to show our country as a country full of goons but in reality these people form very small part of the society. Majority of the doctors love their profession and try their best in treating their patients. In the same way, majority of the patients respect and trust their doctors. But highlighting the negative elements bring a bad name to the whole community and seriously affects the doctor-patient relationship.

Solution:

1. Proper referral system and strengthening rural or

Primary and Secondary Health Care – This point has been given so much importance in this book because implementing this will reduce more than half or even more health care problems.

2. Teaching medical ethics and soft skills to budding doctors at both undergraduate and post graduate level – Actually ethics cannot be taught. They are in built in a person depending upon his/her upbringing and the society where he/she comes from. But still there are ideal things which

should be done in a situation. This is what ethics is all about. Every doctor should learn about medical ethics. In countries where health is topmost priority, there is a separate subject called medical ethics which is taught to undergraduate students.

3. Teaching the patient about how the health system of our country works – Even when you ask educated people in the society that if they know about three tier health system in the country (primary, secondary and tertiary), the answer will be 'NO'

from most of them. So we cannot expect much from uneducated part of the society. Everything which we expect from our society will best come out in the expected way if we teach these things in the school. For example- if a child is never taught in the school that he/she should not litter the surrounding place, then there is very less possibility that he/she will practice the habit of keeping his surroundings clean; no matter how much our government advertises about *'Swach Bharat'*. This person will still spit *'paan'* at public places, throw garbage out on the roads and what not. All this happens because these people have never developed the habit of keeping their country clean.

In nutshell, if we want our people to follow the ideal health system, they must be taught about it right from the schools. There should be a chapter in every school/board curriculum outlining the ideal working of health system in our country. This should not be to overburden students with one more examination question but to make them aware that how important is it to follow the referral system, to teach them the difference between a MBBS/MD/MS doctor and other quacks sitting around.

Problem 3: Frustration of PG students with their subject.

This is problem is on the rise because many doctors choose their specialty depending upon their ranks. This statement holds true especially for top rankers because bottom rankers already have very limited choices but top rankers have every field in front of them. Suppose a student who appeared for post graduate entrance exam got rank in top 10. He likes general Surgery but he sees that the trend these days is that top rankers take Radio diagnosis or Dermatology. So he leaves General Surgery seat and opts for either of the latter fields. But he does not realize that whatever he has chosen at this point, he has to work in that field for the rest of his life (not considering if he goes for IAS or MBA afterwards out of frustration). So choosing your field of interest is very important. It is beneficial for the doctor as well as for his patients.

There is an algorithm which may help medical students in deciding their specialty of choice. There are some other valuable points in it as well. It is

published in Journal of Asian
Medical Students Association.
Do google the 'The Kajal
Algorithm'.

BRAIN DRAIN

There is no denial in the fact that a lot of young talent from India goes abroad and never return back. So we lose many young minds to other countries which are already developed. In health sector there is increasing curiosity to work outside India. All the problems described in previous sections in a way or the other give birth to the idea of practicing medicine abroad. Although there are many hardships which a doctor from developing country needs to face when he tries to get into the health system of developed nations, but he is ready to pass every hurdle just to get out of his own country's health system. This is a sad reality. Following are some of the reasons why Indian doctors want to go abroad-

a) Better quality of life for a doctor in foreign countries

b) More secure jobs

c) More salary

d) Hard work actually pays off in the future

e) Absence or minimal use of alternative medicine which is not proven by medical fraternity

f) Comfortable atmosphere at work place (unlike in India where in some departments or in some hospitals every senior intentionally and un-necessarily wants to make junior's life as hell)

g) More opportunities for research

h) Less burden and hence more personal time

i) Educated patients

j) Advanced hospital facilities (so doctors actually practice protocols which they read in books)

Until and unless whole health system of India is reformed, this brain drain will not stop. The sad story is that there are very few government hospitals which provide quality care to patients (although doctors and staff working there try their best but they have restrictions) and there are many private hospitals which provide best possible care but are too costly for majority of Indian population. So this difference needs to be narrowed down.

MEDICAL TOURISM

India can be a hub of best and affordable medical care in the world if the reforms are brought quickly in the present day health system. India has some of the best doctors in the world who provide best quality and affordable care to the patients. But still very few people can afford this. If foreign money is brought into the country, the prices will automatically reduce for India's native population.

For example, these days only few Indians can afford a liver transplant. But this cost is affordable when compared to expenditure which one has to bear for same surgery in foreign country. If somehow Indian hospitals acquire the trust of other countries and some of its hospitals make a name in the world's best hospitals, then patients will come to India for getting operated because they will get the same quality here at a much cheaper price. This will add to the economy and prices can be reduced for our own population.

THE ROOT CAUSE OF CHAOS

Any problem always has a beginning. Problems just don't arise out of anywhere. Something or the other must have gone wrong at some point of time that we are facing a problem in our present time. Let's figure out what is that one thing in our education system.

When a student clears any entrance examination after 12th standard and gets a seat in a college, it's a great achievement for him/her because finally he will live his dream of becoming what he dreamt of as a child (**provided this was the dream of the student**). The words written in bold have great significance because in India most students are like sheep who just follow the orders and do only what their fellows are doing. The dream of doing something else instead of becoming a doctor/engineer remains with the students and dies with them. It's not their fault. It's not like India has lesser opportunities than developed world. Then where's the problem? Why do Indian students suffer so much? Why do they have to choose among some specified courses?

The only problem is – 'No guidance / counselling'. An average Indian student passes his 10th class exams by the age of 14 – 15 year. Now is the time for him/her to choose the stream he wants to go into. At this age, the mind can't think what is right and what is wrong as a career. A doctor's child wants to go for medical field solely because his dad/mom is a doctor. An engineer's child wants to enter into IIT. Again it is not the fault of these children. They choose these fields because they have never seen other careers. A child from doctor's family has always been in that doctor environment. He has no or very little exposure to life of other careers. Here comes the role of counselling. This student should be counselled about options apart from medical or non-medical field. And he/she should be counselled that there's no shame in going for arts, commerce, economics, business, computers, history, photography, writing, singing, choreography, sports and many other options if you are a doctor's, engineer's, teacher's or for that matter anyone's child.

You have to follow what you like. Obviously you have to take advise from your elders/counselors about what you are about to choose as a career. For example, if you are interested in singing and want to make it as your career but your parents advise you to go for some formal or I can say fixed subjects which other students choose, go for any of these subjects which you like the most and continue taking singing lessons and keep trying your luck by participating in singing competitions. If you are choosing medical as a career, keep singing as your hobby and continue learning and practicing singing. This way you will keep your mind refreshed because probably you like singing more than medicine. And if you are fortunate enough, may be one day you will launch your own album and start your singing career. Now you must be thinking that if singing was what I wanted as a career from the beginning, then why did I choose one of the fixed subject as a career at first on my parent's advice? Remember that your parents are always worried about you and your career more than you yourself are. In today's world, every parent no matter in what field wants the future of their children to be secure. They know that there are too many excellent singers out there who are just struggling with their life. So they are worried that if you don't make it, then what will happen. So they advise you to choose from these fixed fields because in these fixed fields, you will earn something or the other later in life. I am not saying that opting for these fixed fields is compulsory but to make yourself a little bit secure you have to complete your studies in something. But don't worry, you can always and always leave them in between. There is no harm in that. Suppose a person studying engineering but interested in Cricket gets selected in Indian Cricket team, he always has the option to leave engineering, pursue his dream career and never come back to engineering. He had chosen engineering earlier just to make himself a bit secure in life but he continued his passion for cricket.

So the conclusion is: Follow your heart. Take advice from your elders. This is applicable to everyone.

These things will be inculcated in minds of children only and only when there is proper guidance at younger age group. Otherwise what will happen is that a doctor's child interested in singing will opt for medical, give up his dream of becoming a singer, become a doctor, gets frustrated, and harms himself as well as society.

What about those kids whose parents are running a small shop, a road vendor, etc.? These are the kids who need maximum counselling. Even their parents need counselling because they have little idea about career options.

So we have figured out that one thing that leads to chaos in everyone's life i.e. Wrong choice at the beginning.

In conclusion:

Problem – No guidance/counselling of children / parents about changing trends, future prospects, etc.

Solution – A trained counselor/ good teacher who has knowledge about career prospects in every school in India who helps children and parents think together and plan.

At the end, I again emphasize that do what you like, what your heart says. A counselor can only show you all the paths. But at the end it is your decision to choose one or even two paths and then leave one or keep both!

References

a) Rural Health Statistics of India 2012 by Statistics Division, Ministry of Health and Family Welfare, Government of India

b) www.mciindia.org

c) www.fmsc.ac.in – Guidelines for Internship training program